Running with The Sun

Heather J. List

One

She'd been waiting to give him his present for months. She knew exactly what she wanted to get for him and was relentless in the number of times she could bring it up. She'd whisper it in my ear and just to be playful she'd ask him when his birthday was. Two weeks he answered. And the next week, "one more day until I get to open my present!"

"What kind of wrapping paper should I get?" I asked.

She whispered, "Green and yellow, for the Packers. Oh, and a green and yellow bow to go on top." Chloe had the perfectly gift-wrapped package in her head and wouldn't settle for less. "He's *really* gonna love my present."

I smiled and kissed her on the head. I asked Ella if she was ready, but she wasn't. She shook her head and ran for her favorite hiding place—under the piano. I caught her just as she slipped behind the pedals. Put on your jacket, we're going shopping. I knew that shopping wouldn't be enough to compel her out of her hideout, so I thought for a moment and said, "Outside?"

Outside! Outside! Ella loved being outside. It must have come from her father. Every experience I've had outside started off with a pleasant idea of a hike in the woods or a fishing trip with my husband, but they all ended with either a candle full of charred ticks or at least one welt from a beastly insect of Michigan.

Even a family trip to a cabin on Lake Huron turned into a lemon. The cottages were beautiful. They were set up in tiny communities along the shore. Les Cheneaux was well known in Michigan to have both the best fishing and the fewest restaurants. I loved the park, the sand, and the peaceful shore. I even decided to try kayaking to take in the beauty.

I grabbed the kayak from the Tahoe and pushed it into the water. The plastic looked a lot lighter than it was. I heard the water under the kayak as I got in. It made a drumming sound but less harsh. I waved as I pushed off from the beach and set out to discover something, anything. The shore curved into the lake and back again. It was one of the reasons the cabin communities were so private. You couldn't see the adjacent beaches with the natural shoreline. I paddled slowly to take in the homes and the tourists playing on every beach.

I listened to the soft water streaming from the paddles' ends. Each stroke left a ripple in the surface of Lake Huron. I felt small in the lake. There were clouds overhead but I could feel the sun through them. It warmed my face.

After I returned to the beach where we stayed Mona, my boyfriend's mom asked if something was wrong. "No, but is something wrong with my eye? It's itching." 20 minutes later my eye had gone from a mosquito sized lump to an eye swollen shut. Even at the hospital the doctor pulled me aside to ask if it was really a bug. "I wouldn't come to ask for something to stop the reaction if I wasn't having one." I thanked them when I left.

Ella finally put on her jacket. She tested the zipper and smiled at me. She always knew what she should and shouldn't do, but it never stopped her from testing my limits. I didn't mind though. I loved that she had a little spunk behind her eyes. It promised something exciting would always be just a second away. Maybe she'd run after the deer in the yard like her sister had, or she'd pretend to give me a hug and laugh as she tried to bite my chin. Either way, she was perfectly feisty.

Chloe had to stay home from the store. Instead of feisty she was independent and unwavering. She'd make a great CEO, but she has been a very trying 5 year-old. Tonight's battle: cheesy mashed potatoes. No matter how often we promised we wouldn't make her try something she didn't like, and no matter how many prizes and treats we promised she still wouldn't eat them. She'd make herself throw up the microscopic bite of potatoes she put in her mouth before she'd swallow it and admit defeat.

She is smart though. She was three the first time Ryan stepped up to discipline her. Chloe had to sit at the table with us at the family cabin to eat dinner—instead of playing on her own. Chloe thought it was a game. Her best friend was trying to tell her what to do. She didn't even listen to her mom why would she listen to him? She laughed every time she got up from the table and ran off. Ryan was diligent. He'd pick her up and put her right back into the wooden chair. Chloe laughed hysterically when Ryan raised his voice.

After an hour or so of laughter and games Chloe finally figured out that he was serious. He plopped her in the corner next to the pile of wood and old yellowing newspapers. When she realized what was happening, she cried. She didn't just cry like an angry toddler either; she wept. It was the saddest day of her life. Her best friend just yelled at her and made her stand in the corner. The tears ran quietly for few minutes before Ryan rescued her and they walked to the beach. She loved throwing rocks into Lake Gogebic, but I could see she understood. Things were different.

Tonight, Chloe did not win the potato battle but neither did we. She didn't eat the potatoes. Instead she cleaned the house with Ryan until bedtime. She cleared the table, emptied the cold food into the dog's dish, and helped rinse the dishes. She even straightened the living room trying to reestablish the dynamic. You can almost see the wheels turning behind her eyes. She knows exactly what she wants, how to get it, and who to ask. She's only five.

I worked hard on Ryan's present this year too. I even tried to trick him into thinking that I hadn't bought him anything. It backfired and I accidentally hurt his feelings, but he likes surprises, so he tried to smile when I explained why I hid it from him.

Ryan is so worried about everyone else that he won't stop for a second to take care of himself. He chases the girls all night playing monsters, bears, and baseball. I tease him that he needs a boy to play with—then he's sure to mention the nerf guns that he "bought for Chloe" in his closet.

He won't even go fishing. He loves fishing—he used to write for a Michigan fly-fishing magazine. He has a box filled with fuzzies and fishhooks in his office collecting dust. I bought him nice waders, a fishing pole, and a hammock for the cabin. I even told him he had to buy a fishing boat when we were expecting Ella to arrive any day.

I know I make it worse when I try to help. We are buying a

house, a beautiful house, and our real estate broker is just a little older than Ryan with a few boys of his own. He asked Ryan to go fishing and I immediately volunteered him. He was not thrilled with my volunteering—he had plans. He only didn't want to go because I interfered.

Apparently, there is a guy code about making friends that I just don't understand. I think it even involves something about being stupid together. I can see that. Ryan's been planning a man-attack on my new boss for weeks. He was taunted about my being a better fantasy football player than he is. I think it stung a little. Ryan has cautiously asked a few random questions about my boss. What movies does he like, does he have a good sense of humor, and does he wear women's clothing? The last one I came up with on my own, but I bet that just proves Ryan's point—I know nothing about this man-code for friendship.

This year, I bought Ryan a hiking outfit complete with safe hiking sandals that aren't too sandle-ish. I ordered a green short sleeve button up shirt with sweat-wicking technology to keep him cool. I even got him a pair of sandy colored khaki shorts to wear. The shorts he wears are nearly see-through they're so old.

Ryan is a wonderfully kind, loving, fun, and very attractive man so he can pull off anything he wears. But I wanted him to have everything he needed to get outside this year. He hasn't worn them yet, but he says he will when it warms up. He doesn't wear short sleeves until June or something like that.

His birthday came quickly this year. He was a little sad when he woke up that morning. I think birthdays are getting more difficult every year. He's 37. That didn't stop him from getting excited for his presents from the girls though.
Ella picked out the birthday cards. Hers was a monkey that lifted out of a pile of bananas and made loud noises when Ryan opened it. She's almost two so it suited her. She helped wrap her present this year too; 15 plain white undershirts for Daddy. Chloe bought him something I wasn't sure he'd like, an Aaron Rodger's jersey. She wanted all of us to have one.

Ryan likes the Lions, but he is a great dad. He swallowed his pride, put on the jersey, and took a picture with all of us in Rodgers jerseys. He even sent it to his parents to show them he lost the battle with the Packers. Chloe flung her hand in the air and said, I think he will give up on the Lions now. Little stinker.

Ryan and I went to dinner that night at the local steakhouse. We were going to take the girls but they got too tired and crabby, so I called my mom to come watch them for an hour. I could tell she didn't want to, but she came over anyway. She was always so good with the girls. She played just like one of them. I could never get the Barbie's to say the right thing, but my mom could.

Ryan and I were getting dinner ready for them in the kitchen. We were playful as usual. He liked to tease me about dressing up for a simple dinner and I was teasing him about his need to clean and organize everything down to the second. Even the girls' dinner was timed perfectly so that everything was done at the same time—noodles, canned peaches, and corn. I grabbed something from the microwave and felt something strange run down my leg. I ran to the bathroom to hide from Ryan before he saw it.

Just my period. I told myself that I'd change and clean up and I would be ready to go again. I hadn't had my period in months. It wasn't strange to go that long without one, but it was strange for it to start so abruptly and with so much blood. I dug a pad out from the linen closet, cleaned up, and grabbed a new pair of jeans. Ready.

Bye-bye! Chloe grabbed me and hugged me tight before she ran off to the living room to play with grandma again. Ella was a little clingier. She loved Mommy and Daddy. She loved "rocka-rocking" and watching Diego on Nickelodeon. She loved that I bribed her with M&Ms to make time for tying pigtails into her curly hair. "Choc-at!" She didn't like getting her hair done, but she loved chocolate!

Ryan and I left holding hands. In the car he asked why I ran off from the kitchen. I hated having to admit that I was having a period. He laughed. He said he didn't think I even had them anymore. I didn't laugh. I was sore and uncomfortable. So much for my plans for Ryan's birthday.

I was still bleeding heavily when we left for dinner. Since Ryan was on the phone with his parents, I asked him to stop by Walgreens so I could run in. I had an IUD in place, so I shouldn't be pregnant, but I had to be sure. I never bleed that much, and I had to make sure any child I had would be safe—even if I didn't plan it. I bought a two-pack of pregnancy tests and stuffed them into my purse. I told Ryan what I was going to do. He laughed, but it was definitely a nervous laugh. We were quiet on the way to the restaurant.

I slipped into the restroom before we sat at the table. I was scared. I was bleeding so much I knew that even if I was pregnant, I might not be for long. I wiped away the red blood and tried to miss the drips as I was taking the test. I set the test on the toilet paper's container. I stared down into the toilet where red pieces of flesh drifted to the bottom. I imagined that this was nothing. I wasn't pregnant, I wasn't scared, and I certainly wasn't going to get a positive test. But I did.

I wanted to cry but I couldn't. Even though I knew that I may have already lost the baby, I had hope that I was OK. I'd read a book during each of my pregnancies and they discussed, in detail, implantation bleeding. My baby was just implanting into the wall of my uterus where she'd be safe. Or where *he'd* be safe. I had a smile on my face when I thought that I might have a baby boy.

I sat slowly when I reached our booth. Well? Ryan looked nervous. I smiled. I'm pregnant. He laughed, just like he had when I told him about Ella. She was conceived while on birth control pills. I tried not to blame myself for the surprise but when you tell anyone you got pregnant on the pill, they roll their eyes and say, sure you did. But I did. I tried to convince myself I had taken the pill at the wrong time one day, or that maybe it was something I ate that made it ineffective. But I was excited for Ella, just like I was excited for this one. It didn't matter whether the children were planned or not.

After having Chloe, and the ordeal we went through together, I knew that no matter what situation a child came into the world—they were perfect. I knew that I would love them and that everything would be fine because I could hold that tiny baby and the tears would fall down my cheeks and onto a perfect, tiny child. I could love completely, unselfishly, unconditionally, and plow through anything difficult because I had someone to care for and love.

And the baby loved me the same way. Even when Chloe is angry at me, she still tries to cuddle her way out of her punishment. She'll give me a kiss when I cry or a joke when I'm tired. She tucks me in on the couch if I didn't make it to the bed and pushes my hair out of my face if I don't open my eyes. I don't open my eyes on purpose. I just let her take care of me the way I did with her. Her fingernails are full of dirt and her nail polish is breaking off, but those tiny sticky fingers slide across my forehead and it makes me feel loved. She even has a sideways smile while she stares at me.

Ryan ordered a tall beer. I ordered a Diet Pepsi—no ice. The server could tell something weird was happening at the table but tried to stay out of it. Ryan couldn't stop laughing. He said I was super fertile and that we should've known. I even felt relieved. At least we know that Ella was not my fault now, nothing would have prevented her arrival! We laughed. Ryan was playful again, are you sure you didn't plan this? I was sure. I wasn't sure of what to do next. I was still bleeding. We ordered steak and talked, but the conversation grew quiet as we realized the baby needed to be checked on right away. We decided that I should go to the emergency room that night after dinner. I felt sick to my stomach.

They all stared at me when I walked in. I waited for them to ask what I needed, or why I was crying, or send me to a bed. They didn't. They just stared at me and waited. There was a steaming dinner lying on the bed behind them. The nurses must be trying to have a break. I felt bad. I thought about leaving and just coming back to the clinic in the morning, but I'd do anything for this baby. "I need to be seen." The tears gushed behind the words and I pulled my hands into the sleeves of Ryan's sweater. It was forest green, a little ratty and torn, but it smelled like him.

What's going on? I didn't know what to say, but the words flung from my mouth between the heaving breaths. "I have an IUD, I'm pregnant, and I'm bleeding." The nurse asked me to follow her and had me lay down in a room with a door. They shut the door and I was alone.

The walls were plain white with a shiny gleam. They probably needed paint they could clean in case of a mess. Just before the walls met the ceiling there was a line of wallpaper trim. Fawns, raccoons, and small animals pranced across the walls. I could put cute wallpaper in the baby's room. But not this paper. This paper was faded and boring.

The nurse came in and checked my blood pressure, my heart, and my lungs. She said the first thing to do was to take a blood test to make sure I was pregnant. She was right. There was so much blood on the pregnancy test I had taken maybe the second line appeared because the blood stained it.

The cart rolled up outside of the door. She introduced herself and said she'd be quick. She congratulated me on the pregnancy. I couldn't look at, or think about, what she was doing. I trailed off. There were so many things I wanted to look forward to. How would I tell the girls? I could buy them new shirts. Ella's could say I'm the big sister, and Chloe's could say I'm the biggest sister. Or I could buy and wrap three toys. They'd each open theirs and ask who the third gift was for.

Just a little pinch here. I hate when they say that. It's never just a little pinch. I told myself to breathe in, breathe out. The nurse said I had to breathe for the blood to come out. Breathe in, breathe out. Don't talk about the blood. All done, you can look now. I looked, but snapped my eyes shut again. They took so much. I'll wait, I told her, until it's all gone and covered. She laughed again. When everything was clean, I opened my eyes again and she left. There was still a spot of blood on the bed. I felt sick again and rolled over to my side.

Just as I closed my eyes my phone buzzed. Ryan wanted to know how I was. I was fine, just waiting for the test to come back.

The nurse said it'd be at least an hour. Ryan wanted to come to the hospital to sit with me, but he had the girls. I told him I was fine, and he didn't need to worry, that I'd call if I needed him.

Ryan called a friend of his. Curtis was a single colleague of Ryan's who had made a or himself in our area. I am not sure I would have called him to babysit, but in this situation I understood. When Ryan arrived at the hospital, he thought I might be upset about Curtis so before I said anything, he explained that Curtis was great with his nieces and he'd be fine with the two sleeping girls at home. I was just glad Ryan came. He slid into the cot with me and he said he had faith in my fertility. His sense of humor is awkward, but it was just what I wanted to hear.

The hour was so long, but the doctor finally came in. He was in his fifties with glasses. were still cuddled in the cot when he said, you are definitely pregnant. You're going to be a family. We smiled; we were already a family. He must have thought since we were still cuddling together with our iPhones that we were young and childless. But we weren't childless, and we weren't that young.

"The IUD has to come out as soon as possible." I already knew that. I read that the IUD can cause serious pregnancy complications if left in—but that all depended on how far along I was. "You're four to five weeks." That's still plenty of time to get it out. He made an appointment with my doctor for the next day and said, "we don't do that here." I wondered what they could do here. He sent me home with a stack of information on threatened miscarriages.

Ryan and I drove home. I cried. I didn't know if I should be excited for a baby or sad for a loss. I climbed into bed and heard Ryan and Curtis talking in the living room. Curtis never knew when to leave, but it sounded like Ryan was talking to him about the baby. Maybe Ryan needed Curtis as much as I needed Ryan. I fell asleep on his side of the bed.

The next morning, I went to my doctor's office. The nurse asked if anyone was with me, I said no. We walked quietly to the ultrasound room. She took the vital signs, congratulated me, and said the doctor would be right back. They came back together. I was crying again, and I could tell they felt bad for me. I just wanted the baby to be OK, I loved the baby. I wanted to make sure that removing the IUD wouldn't hurt the baby.

A little cold here. A transvaginal ultrasound was a very uncomfortable position to be in. I was still bleeding a little, and I had two people staring inside of me. I'd do anything for the baby, though, even humiliating things like peeing in a cup and shoving plastic tools into myself.

The doctor studied the screen for a second. There was a gestational sac, and a growth from an ovary—the corpus luteum he explained. The baby pregnancy was still there, and the IUD looked like it was low enough not to hurt the baby, but he couldn't promise that it wouldn't cause a miscarriage. The best chance for the baby was to take it out.

I laid back, prayed asking God to put his hand over the baby, and cried. All done. I carefully sat up and lost control of myself. The doctor explained that the IUD came out clean and that if I lost the baby, it was nothing that we did that day. It was hard to believe. He also set up a lab test for me on Monday to see if I would still be pregnant. If the HCG, human chorionic gonadotropin, levels were going up, I was pregnant. If they were going down, then I lost the baby. I cried all the way home.

I stood up to get out of the Jeep and felt the same trickle I felt the night before. I ran to the bathroom and blood ran out into the toilet. I cried and begged God not to take the baby. I thought about the positive test and how happy I was. I remembered the test for each of my daughters, and then I opened my eyes again. I was still there in the bathroom covered in salty tears. I grabbed a washcloth, soaked it in warm water and cleaned up. Before I flushed, I saw bits of tissue again in the water, like at the restaurant. I cried. I didn't know if I could flush. The tears hit the water and I pulled the lever.

My bed never felt colder than when I got in that day. I couldn't stop crying. My pillow was wet on both sides before I realized I wouldn't be able to sleep like this. I walked to the kitchen, unplugged the iPod dock, and crawled back into our bed. I needed to connect with the baby. I wanted to sleep knowing that the baby was OK. I plugged my iPhone into the dock and searched Pandora for a station I could listen to. Religious, yoga, country? I couldn't decide, but I knew I needed something without words. Relaxation radio.

Something beautiful filled my ears. I could hear a river, trees, and a piano. I put my hand over my stomach and closed my eyes. I imagined a place I thought God might let me see my baby. I flipped through the pages of my journal in my head.

I remembered a moment last spring on Lake Superior. It was still cold, but I always feel the urge to honor my annual pilgrimage to the lake. The road was long and winding. The houses got further and further apart as we got closer to the lake. Ella had been to this beach before, but this was the first time she'd see and touch it. The last time we were here she was just a squirming little baby excited when the water touched my swollen belly.

The earth on the beach wasn't sandy, but instead was covered in rocks. Pale blue and grey sandstones were piled high on the beach. Through the winter, the rocks were carried by the lake to shore where the harsh winter winds threw them onto the icy shore where they stayed trapped until spring. When the wind relaxed into to a warm breeze the ice melted, and like the glaciers that created the lake, they left behind the rocks from winter.

Chloe loves sandstones, they're her favorite. But it was just Ella, Ryan and I that day. We walked up to the edge of the water. The sound of the thick waves caught my breath and took it away with them. The rocks moved under our feet with every step. Balancing was hard. I knelt for a minute and I remember watching the water rushing beneath our feet under the rocks toward the lake. The rolling hills behind us sent the groundwater to the beach. It swirled when it hit the water and disappeared.

Ryan held his hand out for me, and I leaned on him for a moment watching the waves and the sun melt together. We decided to get married on the beach that day… when it got warm enough.

My eyes were still closed, and my face was still wet, but the tears had stopped. I opened them to see that I was still in our bed with the music. I didn't want to get up yet. I was afraid of what might fall out if I stood up. So, I closed my eyes again.

~*~

The beach was still beautiful, but it was warmer this time. The sun was high, and the beach was sandy. It was the same beach as last spring, but this time the sandstones were further back, and there was a wide line of sand between the rocks and the water. There wasn't a path back to any road, or trail to follow. It was just the sand, the water, and a dark green forest behind me. Behind us.

I was lying on a reclined white beach chair. I was wearing a blue bikini on and bare feet. A white towel was tied around my waist and hung just over the edge of the chair. My baby was lying on my stomach with its head cuddled into my shoulder. Light fuzzy hair, closed eyes, and a white blanket over its lower back and legs. I didn't even know if there was a diaper.

The sun was warm, but it was not hot out. It was comfortable. The waves came in and left, the trees continued their soft song behind us, and the baby's breath warmed my shoulder with every rise and fall of its chest. I love you, baby.

I tucked my chin next to the baby's head on my shoulder. Baby's nose faced the East and I looked north toward the water. I could feel the baby's breathing. Up then down again. I could feel the moist spot on my shoulder where baby's breath warmed it. I could feel the baby squirming in my arms to get comfortable then sighing a breath of relief and sleeping again.

I tucked a pillow under my right arm to relieve the weight of the baby under my arm. Perfect. I had a sun hat on, but I still looked up and thanked the sun for the warmth it was providing. I smiled at the blue sky, and I rubbed baby's back. The sand started to rustle under us with the breeze, but even when it settled under my legs, I didn't mind. I just made sure baby's face was protected from getting sun in its eyes.

Sitting in the chair, I thought about Chloe's infancy. She was tiny. She was 17 inches tall and 5 pounds 11 ounces when she was born. She was warm and wrapped in pink before she was whisked off with her doctors to make sure she was ok. I sat in the delivery room alone for nearly two hours before I got to hold her again.

She was squirming in my arms crying for milk. I tried to breastfeed her. I didn't know what I was doing. The nurse came in to help me. Chloe was soothed by my breast even though the milk wasn't ready for her. She quieted and drifted to sleep in my arms. She had never met me, but she loved me. She was nestled into the nook of my elbow. She comforted herself with her hands resting on her cheeks near her ears. She was so tiny.

Chloe slept through the first few days. She only woke to cry for Mommy. The nurses would call me right away if she woke up because she'd cry so loud, she would wake up the other babies. The neonatal ICU was quiet. They kept the lights low for the newborns. They had soft rocking chairs at each station for the mothers to hold the tiny children. Chloe was the biggest, and healthiest of them. I was so lucky to have her in my arms. She was perfect.

Ella was 21 inches tall and 7 pounds 5 ounces when she was born. She was not tired. Mommy was tired after nearly 12 hours of labor and pain, but Ella was awake. She sucked on her hands and stared at Daddy. She loved him. Then Grandpa took her, and she stared at him. She loved him. Mommy held her for a long time but instead of staring she began looking for milk. She was hungry when she was born. I laughed and slipped my bra down to let her suckle. She knew just what to do. She even started crying again a few minutes later when there wasn't milk for her. Poor thing. She went back to sucking her hands and making the cutest sounds. Ooh and hu-hu, hu-hu. The world was new and interesting. She stayed awake for four hours before she finally gave into sleep.

Here, on the warm beach, I didn't have a delivery. I was just holding my baby safely under the sun that hung over us. I wondered how things could be any more perfect. I thought about his eyes. What color were they? I picked him up and tucked in into my elbow. I tried to see his eyes, but I couldn't. They were closed.

That's OK, I could see them later. I put him back up onto my shoulder and closed my eyes with him. The sun was so warm.

~*~

The door slammed and I heard Ryan sneak into our room. I opened my eyes. The room was dark, but the sun was peering through the small space between the curtains. Before I laid in bed, I sent him a text saying that I needed him home. I didn't know how I could stop crying without him. He said he'd come to see me but that he could only stay for an hour. He stared at me. I could tell he was trying to see what I felt. I let myself cry again with my head tucked into his chest. We closed our eyes and laid sideways on our bed together.

I must have fallen asleep because it was only a second later that the door slammed again, and I could hear voices. The girls were home. I could hear Ella, Where's Mommy? Ryan tried to quiet them with snacks, TV, and whispers. They just wanted their Mommy.

I didn't know if I could stand. I sat at the edge of the bed for a minute listening. Choc-at? I smiled, stood, and walked to the bathroom. This time, there was no new blood. I cleaned up again. *Three more days until I'll know where my baby is.* I took a cold cloth and covered my face. I tried to put makeup on. I don't remember if it made me look any better, but the girls hugged me when I came down the hall. They are so precious.

We sat down to dinner. Chloe reminded us to pray. Her favorite:

Come Lord Jesus be our guest, and let thy gifts to us be blessed. Amen. Appa, Leaper, Father, Amen!

Ella clapped. She loved the last part. She even tried to say it now. I don't even know what it means, but Ryan's family says it after every prayer. Ella just likes to fold her hands and clap. She'll understand better when she gets older.

Chloe understands God better than most adults. Adults falter and search, they question and are either all one way or another.

Children don't over analyze faith. Chloe understands love, fear, heaven, and faith better than we do. She came home from daycare one day and told me about her friends.

Trinity Childcare is a Lutheran based daycare. Chloe colors religious drawings throughout her day, sings with the pastor, and hears bible stories. Her friends heard a story about heaven and how God saves people. She said they thought God lived in heaven. *God is in your heart you know.* She said she wanted to go to heaven for a day. Of all the things to be confused over, and to question, Chloe understood the most important piece of God from the beginning. *God is in your heart you know.*

It took me years to find God. I believed in God, but I wanted to feel God. I searched everywhere, churches, mountains, water, ancient cultures, other religions, and the bible. It took having my first daughter to see God for the first time. Finding that even sitting on my rocking chair in my tiny apartment God was with me. When I learned that I was having Ella, I was scared. I didn't know what would happen. I went for a walk and felt the sun on my cheek. *God is in your heart you know.* Chloe was right.

We talked about our day at the dinner table. Ella covered herself in mashed potatoes and Chloe talked about how she didn't like math but that she was really good at it. She said she was bored at school because it was too easy, and she just wanted to play. I couldn't help but laugh a little. She's just like me; a little feisty but soft on the inside. She helped clear the table and we did family cuddle time on the couch. Ella wanted to rock so Daddy took her to the rocking chair and Chloe, and I sat on the couch. I fell asleep with her sitting next to me.

The weekend was a blur. It was a combination of crying and hopeful thinking. Ryan and I talked about praying together, and the color the baby's room would be. We were buying a house with three bedrooms, so we decided to have Chloe and Ella share when baby moved out of our room. We talked about when the baby was due and if we'd try again if we'd lost the baby.

~*~

I returned to the beach every time I closed my eyes. Sunday night I needed the beach more than before. I was nervous for the blood test in the morning. I laid in bed while the girls and Ryan were still playing in the living room. I turned my relaxation radio on. The tears fell for a while at first. Then the sun dried them off. Baby was sleeping in a crib on the beach. The crib was covered by a white outdoor canopy. There were cloth walls preventing the sand from getting into Baby's bed. I walked through the slit in the cloth. The canopy was sturdy, but the walls were slowly waving in the breeze.

I looked down at the sleeping child. Baby's hair was still fuzzy, and the white blanket was still wrapped around him. He was lying on his back turned slightly toward his left arm. He still had the reflex to protect himself from rolling over. His belly button peered over the blanket. I reached down and swept Baby into my arms. He was warm but he still curled up against my shoulder like he had last time.

We sat in the chair for a while. I still wanted to see his eyes. I grabbed the quilt from the canopy and laid it out over the sand. I carefully laid him down on the blanket. He squirmed a little. I laid next to him in the sand. I put my arm behind him to protect him. He felt me near and started to look for my breast. I scooted closer to him and untied my top. He was very hungry.

He tugged for a while before he let go and slept beside me. I knew he wouldn't wake up today, not after I had fed him. I kissed his forehead and I watched his chest rise and fall one more time. Then I closed my eyes beside him for a nap. The sun kept us warm as we laid on the quilt in the sand.

~*~

Ryan shook me to open my eyes. "You have to wake up, Alex." I knew I had to wake up, but I wasn't ready to. I knew it would be cold outside that early. There was still frost on the grass in the middle of April. Last year we still had snow at this time, so I shouldn't complain, but it was so much warmer in bed.

We got the girls dressed and ready for school. I bribed both girls with gummy worms to do their hair. I got one ponytail into Chloe's hair and pigtails into Ella's. Chloe said that kids her age don't wear pigtails anymore. She showed me her socks. There was one blue and one pink. I asked her why and she laughed. I couldn't find the other blue sock, so I made crazy socks! That made sense to me. She hopped on the bus and went to her kindergarten class.

I wrestled Ella into the car. She'd rather be outside than in the car. She didn't like the straps, the jacket, the sounds, or leaving home. I usually had to wait a minute or so for her to stop trying to get out before I could buckle her. She would twist herself around stand up in the chair and look over the back of the seat to the trunk. She just laughed when she'd get that far. She'd tighten her tiny fingers around the head rests and if she managed to do that, I'd have to pry her fingers off before I could get her buckled. The trick was to not let her turn around. It was much harder to do than it sounds.

When we arrived at daycare and she said, Play? Play! She knows that daycare is fun, and that she has friends who wait for her. I lifted her over the toddler room's gate and set her down. She was always a bit cautious when first entering the room. She wasn't sure who was going to be crabby, crazy, or silly. Every day she takes a few minutes to examine the situation before she'd get too close to anyone. If any of the boys started to yell, she'd hide behind my leg while I hung her jacket and bags on her hook. She had a hook with her name printed on a colored sheet of paper taped just above it.

Sitting in the waiting room was hard. The lab was busy, and I was third in line. When they finally called me in, I couldn't watch. The doctor will call you by the end of the day. I thanked her and wandered out of the hospital. Only a few more hours.

When the phone rang at work I ran out of the office to the back lot. I froze. The doctor said that my levels were going up. Thank God! But, he said, they are not going up as quickly as I expected them to. He told me to be cautiously optimistic. It was better news than I expected so I called Ryan and told him. He still seemed concerned, but we were excited that we'd made it that far.

I drove two blocks to my house and knelt thanking God. *Even if I can't have this baby, I know you will take good care of him, but I want to do that. Thank you for giving me this baby. I will do anything to make sure he gets here safely.* I cried. I was so grateful for the baby that I was excited. I was finally letting myself be excited.

Another 10 days until my ultrasound to see the baby's heartbeat. At work that day I couldn't concentrate. I let myself look in the mirror and I saw a pregnant woman for the first time. I searched for names for the baby. I wanted to be humble and thank God for the gift of this baby. I searched thousands of names and decided that Nathaniel John List for a boy and Anastasia Lyn List for a girl. Ryan and I met at home for dinner—he liked the names. We let ourselves dream about finishing the attic at the new house, and what colors we'd paint it. We talked about getting a van to fit everyone comfortably into a car. We thought about the new things we'd have to buy and how much we'd spend on the baby before December. December 21st was my due date. We decided that this would be the last baby. Three was perfect for us.

I climbed into bed with Ryan that night. He snuggled close and I set my hand over my belly. I don't know why I'd set my hand there. I couldn't feel Baby yet. I wasn't growing very quickly. But for some reason each time I've been pregnant, my hand sits comfortably just under my belly button. I was holding my baby. I was protecting him. It reminded me of the first appointment to remove the IUD. I cringed and switched my thoughts to the prayer. God please put your hand over this baby to protect him. I closed my eyes and let myself imagine the music from my iPod. I didn't need to turn it on that night.

~*~

The piano danced through my head. I loved the piano. I thought about getting out of bed to play for a while, maybe write something beautiful for Baby. I wanted the sound of my playing to show him how much I enjoyed my time with him near the water. I could hear the notes that would sound like the water under the kayak. And the timing that could sound like the breeze quickening then slowing to a halt and letting go of the sand. The sand would fall back to the earth and be still again.

I could make the music heave to the climax where my baby would open his eyes. I wondered if they were blue, like mine. They must be blue; he has light hair. I read that most babies are born with blue eyes and they change during the first year. My son must have blue eyes.

I walked over to the canopy and reached down to the sleeping baby. He was perfect. He was starting to develop little rolls of skin over his wrists. Each of my daughters were round at this age. I would scold anyone who told me my babies were chunky or fat, but they were right. My babies were fat. I made good milk for them. I thought I should feed him, but I didn't want him to get burned. We'd spent so much time in the sun over the last few days that we probably needed to stay in the shade. I walked over to the sandy wicker chair under the canopy and sat with him.

I tried to wake him by brushing my finger over his cheek. He opened his eyes. His eyelashes were long and dark. A little crease formed under each brow bone, and his sparkling blue eyes stared up at me for the first time. I felt warm tears trickling down my cheeks. He was so beautiful. His hand curled up next to his ear and he began searching for my breast. I held him close and gently rocked myself back and forth for him while he drank.

When he finished a little drop of milk slid across his face and into his hair. I should probably rinse his hair with the lake water, but I decided to let him sleep. I set him down in his crib and stepped out to move the quilt. I dragged it across the sand to the shade near the trees. Maybe I'd sleep next to him. I pulled him from his crib again and laid him next to me on the blanket. He slept so soundly. I rubbed his back for a minute before I drifted off to sleep. *Nathaniel, thank you for spending today with me.*

~*~

Ryan had baseball practice today. He is the head coach for a team of nine and ten-year-olds. He was so excited when he was called by the league and told he had a team. He tried so hard to hold his smile back, but he couldn't. I hadn't seen him so excited since he opened the cabin for the summer last year.

Every year Ryan and his grandma's boyfriend call each other to schedule the date for the cabin opening. Junior is in his 80s and mostly supervises Ryan's work. But together they start the pump house, check the electric, mow the lawn, and clean out the dead flies and mice. I'm not even sure what else is a part of the opening, but I assume it involves beer, chewing tobacco, and talking about the weather and the fish. Ryan always takes his fishing pole, but I don't remember if he's brought any fish home.

When he'd come home, he'd talk about all the work they did and how tired he was and wonders out loud why he volunteers to do it. Because he loves it, I tell him. He won't admit that he loves it. He won't admit that he counts the days before the opening, or that he's been organizing his fishing equipment for two weeks. But he wouldn't let me know he loved baseball this much either. He is a man's man. I love that about him.

Ella and I stayed home while he was at practice. She slept for two hours. I had time to think for two hours. I sat on the rocking chair for a while in silence. The rocking chair faces the patio door so I could see the backyard and the animals. A few deer walked through. We have an apple tree that is on the verge of blooming but hasn't yet.

I've been waiting to see the new fawns but there haven't been any of them either. It should only be a few more weeks. I thought about the day we moved into this house, and how sad we'll be when we move out again. I thought about the room here that would have been Nathaniel's and how it's just an office that never gets used. The girls use it to watch movies—the movie room. The yard is green with wildly growing grass and dandelions. The patio is concrete with cracks and a hole. The old swing set was given to us when we moved here. Ryan's neighbors from his last house gave it to him when they bought their new one. They even helped us haul it to the trailer. It's rusting in the yard now. We left it out all winter. We will buy a new one this summer —after we move.

The baby swing is still hung out there too. Ryan's parents brought it up to us last summer after our wedding. Ella was almost one and just learning to walk. Mona thought it would be fun to push her on the swing while Ryan and I spent the weekend together in Minneapolis. We had our wedding on the beach in Silver City Michigan. It was early on Friday morning, but it was already more than 70 degrees. The sand was hot, the sun was hot, and the seagulls were out. I didn't care. Ryan looked amazing in his black suit. I wore a white, single strapped informal wedding dress. My bare shoulders burned in the sun. I still cried when I held Ryan's hands. He smiled through the entire ceremony and I cried. I was so happy in that moment. My daughters and our parents were guests. It was all about Ryan and me finding each other. He proposed in that spot the year before.

The chair was uncomfortable, but I didn't know what else to do. I decided I'd take a nap but first I walked to the bathroom. I was nervous to use the bathroom since the emergency room. The doctor described what a miscarriage would look like. Bleeding, clots, and tissue. My back would start to hurt with cramping. I didn't feel any of the pain, but I didn't want to be surprised either. I would pray before I walked into the bathroom. Please God, protect my baby.

I reclined the chair, tucked myself under my blanket, and closed my eyes. The tears were always right at the corner of my eyes. I couldn't turn them off. I let the tears fall onto my pillow while I walked to the beach. My baby was waiting for me.

~*~

Hello there. What do you say we go for a walk today? I

tucked my hand behind Nathaniel's head and laid him against my shoulder. His eyes opened revealing their blue innocence. I love you. He's so little. His head stayed comfortably on my shoulder while we walked into the trees. The river was flowing gently down to the lake carving the sand. It was beautiful. The birds were singing to us though I couldn't see them when I looked up. The sun was high and created glowing pieces of warm earth. I found a large oak tree near the river's edge, but not too close. I leaned back and felt the cool bark against my skin. Nathaniel just watched the movement around us. The water, the leaves, and Mommy.

We could still see the sand from where we sat. The shade felt nice. He wasn't hungry but I thought it would be nice to feed him while we were sitting here. I lowered him from my shoulder, and he watched me for a minute. His eyes soaked in my face and my hair. His hand grasped my thumb. He tried to pull it up to his mouth, but I wanted him to eat so I waited. He squirmed a little. His feet kicked up and down and his hands would search for something to hold. His lips were peach, and his tongue wiggled behind them. He was so beautiful. *Even if I never hold you while I'm awake, I am so glad God gave us this time together*. He turned his head and began tugging. I could feel his body relax as he comforted himself. Mine did too.

I leaned my head back against the tree and stared up into the blue sky. The sun was bright but not bright enough to make me look away. The world was perfect here. The sky was as blue as my child's eyes, and the trees were so tall. How could I want to go back?

I looked down from the sky and out into the forest. It didn't look dark anywhere. The trees were spaced just right so that enough sun could reach the soil and the leafy plants on the forest's floor to make for an enchanted retreat. Ryan and I often debated which forests were more beautiful. I tried to explain that the rustic, unmanaged forests of the Upper Peninsula were the perfect forests because they were natural, and untouched. I would know, I'd tell him, I explored them daily while I was a child. I lived 7 miles from the U.P. into Wisconsin, but they were the same. The Penokee

Range bluffs that protected us from the harsher weather of central Wisconsin were the same bluffs that protected the U.P. The forests must be the same.

I loved that when I walked through the forest I had to step over fallen logs, dense underbrush, and boulders that protruded from the moist forest floor. I'd even take yard scissors to cut my way through, I was a child adventurer.

The ticks were horrible. I'd come home with so many ticks, that my mom would march me straight into the bathroom to check. We'd light a candle and pick them off one by one. The worst tick was in my ear. They had to smoke him out. I threw him into the candle myself. The wildlife in our forests were fantastic. I saw blue herons along the spring-fed Weber Lake, mountain lions, bears, coyotes and wolves. All were so natural and rustic—I felt like I was one of them. We were surviving the wilderness together.

Ryan said that the sandy forests of the Lower Peninsula were easier to enjoy. The forest floors were clear. You didn't have to dodge thorny underbrush or boulders. You only had to avoid the trees. I thought about the uprooted trees I'd seen along US 31. The wind must've run quickly through the trees knocking them over. But he was probably right. The openness of the forests there were easier to navigate. I bet they were like this forest. Not as warm or calm, but beautiful and inviting.

Nathaniel's lips slowly slipped from my breast. He was still suckling. A few drops of milk rolled off the corner of his mouth and into his hair. I stood and walked to the edge of the river, swept my hand through the cool water, and wiped away the trail. I dunked my hand one more time and wet the back of his hair. Now it won't get sticky.

I walked with him carefully back to the canopy. The crib was ready for him. I laid him down and spread his blanket over him. I thought he could use a little nap. I sat in the wicker chair and closed my eyes. I listened to the waves wetting the sand, the sand brushing the cloth of the canopy, and the tiny breaths coming from the crib beside me.

~*~

Buttercup started barking. I sat up and ran to the bathroom to clean my face. I used a cold washcloth, eyeliner, and a little cherry lip balm. I brushed my hair, took a breath, and casually walked out. Ryan was home. I asked him about his practice. He walked over to me and hugged me. Are you OK? I said yes. I was OK. He smiled and said practice was hard and that he was sore. He went over his schedule for the next two weeks and wanted me to know he didn't like coaching, that it was going to be a big-time commitment. I smiled with him but not because he was coating the truth—that as a man he can't let himself be excited—but because I loved him.

Ryan and I decided to wake Ella. Chloe was at her dads for the weekend and wouldn't be home until Sunday night. We ran to Ella's room fighting over who would "save her" from her bed. She stood up, already awake, and smiled. Mama! Ryan picked her up, tickled her belly, and kissed her a few times. She giggled every time Daddy would raise her up over his head and kiss her belly.

I picked her up from Ryan and gave her a big hug. Her tiny, almost two-year-old hand patted me on the arm. She sat back and smiled at me. She had most of her teeth now. They had wide spaces between each of them, but they were all there. Her hair is curly like her dad's. It is medium brown and tied into pigtails. They were already starting to fall out, but I loved her hair a little messy. It suited her. I set her down and she took a few steps, looked back at us with a grin, and took off running down the hall. Ryan chased her making monster noises and tickled her on the floor. I went to the kitchen to make her lunch. She must be hungry by now.

The room was swirling. "Sissy! Hi Sissy!" Buttercup was barking, and a loud truck was parked in our driveway. Chloe was home. Her dad carried her to the door, sleeping on his shoulder. He set Chloe down and she sleepily smiled at Ella, "Hi Ella." Her cheeks were pink. Her eyes still had little crusts in each corner. Hi Mommy, Hi Ryan. We missed her.

Hi Sissy! I had bought Chloe two new sets of pajamas while she was gone. She wondered into the kitchen with Ryan to talk to him. Ella followed. He asked about her day and if she had fun. Chloe always had so much to say when she came home. Chloe admired Ryan. She wanted to be a teacher like him, play outside with him, do yard work with him, and watch their show together in our bedroom—without Mommy. I love that they are so close.

I waited and watched from the living room. When Chloe came in to sit down, I told her there was a surprise on her bed in her room. I had cleaned her room for her over the weekend sorting the Polly pockets from the Barbie dolls, and the books into their individual shelves.

The first set of pajamas was a t-shirt with a dog listening to music. The music notes sparkled, and the dog was wearing sunglasses. Chloe called them shades. The second set was a tank top with frilly shoulders and shorts. They were silky and had animals on them. They also had sparkles.

Both Chloe and Ella are princesses with distinct styles. Chloe is my artist. She loves music, painting, drawing, and dancing. She is a wonderful artist and singer. Chloe can draw better than most ten-year-olds. I secretly hope that she'll pursue art as she gets older, but I don't want to push her or even let her know what I want.

Artists like Chloe, come pre-packaged complete with an attitude. Every morning she'll ask me to pick out her clothes for her. And every morning, she will not wear one piece of clothing I set out. I once asked her why she has me pick them out at all. She started laughing and said I don't know, 'cause I don't want to. But you never wear anything I pick? I know, I just like that you help me. Maybe she did, but all I was helping with was to show her what not to wear to school that day. It makes her happy, though, so I do it anyway.

Ella is the cuddly, fun-loving, thinker. Ella is still very young, but you can see when she stops to study something. She also loves to dance, but not because it's artistic, but because she likes to shake her butt and stand on her head looking at me through her legs.

She also likes to cuddle, but she might grow out of that. Ryan and I fight over the cuddle time because we are afraid it won't last much longer. She's been laying on the couch next to us for the last week or so to fall asleep. We are probably planting a horrible issue for bedtime later, but it's so cute that we haven't been able to stop ourselves from letting her.

Chloe put on the sparkly music pajamas and did her model walk out into the kitchen. Oh, Ryan. He turned and said she looked beautiful. She ran off to try the others on for dinner. We sat together and talked about everything. Chloe likes to ask Ryan about stories when he was young. Ryan loves it but won't admit it. He tells a few of the same stories over and over and Chloe loves it. One involves a crazy dog hopping through a corn field and the others are about Grandpa Fred, or Grandma Mona.

Ella's favorite thing about dinner is her mess. She loves to feed the dog, squish her food together, show Mommy her chewed food on her tongue, and pick boogers for Daddy. She is one gross little toddler.

The girls needed a bath, so I started the water. We still had the baby bath from Ella in the corner of the bathroom. I thought about her duckies in that tub, and how wet the carpet was every time she started to splash. I tucked the baby tub into the linen closet and called for the girls. They were half stripped before they even came around the corner.

Ella leaned over the edge to put her hands in the running water. Chloe turned around to shake her bare butt at me. I pinched it and she squealed. Ella tried to climb in, so I lifted her up and over the tile. She loved the water just like when she was in my belly at the beach. She would get so excited to play in it. Chloe liked to play in the water but hated it getting in her face. I didn't like it either.

Three more days until my next ultrasound. I tucked each of the girls into bed and while Ryan was grading papers, I searched websites for photos of ultrasounds at 7-8 weeks gestation. There were thousands of sites willing to share their photos of babies. I saw the four-week ultrasound was just a gestational sac, the five week had a yolk-sac, and the six week had a baby. The seven-week ultrasound would have a baby's heartbeat. I played one from the internet and watched the little pumping of what it named a primitive heart. *No heart is primitive.*

I searched what ultrasounds of twins would look like, so I knew what to look for on Thursday. They showed two babies in one gestational sac, two sacs with two babies, and even three babies! I hoped there was more than one baby. Ryan only wanted one more child, but I secretly could have ten babies and love them all. If there were two, then we'd have four children. It was wishful thinking, though.

I started to search my HCG levels. More than 3000 on a normal scale was high for four weeks. I must've been five weeks at the emergency room. And on the Monday after I was at 3900 so even though it wasn't going up fast enough, it still went up by 30%. The doctor wanted to see a 50% increase, but 30% was close. I looked at the charts again. If I was really 4 weeks in the emergency room, then I might have two. I checked the ultrasound photographs of twins again.

Ryan came over to the couch to watch a movie with me. I closed my computer then I kissed him and rested my head on his lap. Ryan never argued with me falling asleep on him because it meant that he could watch a man movie with explosions, fighting, and machines. Every man needed an outlet for the untamed instinctive creatures that we are. A part of our environment is innately built into us. Being human requires an understanding of ourselves and embracing our nature. Machine guns and fire help Ryan to do that.

~*~

The beach was still warm. The sun seemed lower for the first time. Maybe Nathaniel and I would experience our first night together. The sun hung orange in the sky touching the tops of the trees behind us. It wouldn't come tonight, but soon. I walked into the canopy and watched him breathe for a minute. His chest expanded with every breath he took, and he made a little sound when he let the air out again. He almost sighed with every breath. I noticed a second crib, but I couldn't see anything inside of it. I didn't walk over to it either. I scooped Nathaniel up into my arms and walked over to our chair. I almost sat, but I needed to know if there were two children.

Inside the canopy I looked down into the second crib. There was another baby. This baby had dark brown hair and was a little plumper than Nathaniel. Her hands were folded across her chest with her elbows at either side. She had little indents where dimples might form if she smiled. I couldn't see her chest moving but she had a darker blanket. I carefully picked her up too. Nathaniel turned his head to look at her then laid his ear against my chest. She was sleeping. Two warm babies to hold.

I walked over to our chair and tucked a pillow under each elbow. Each infant had a cheek pressed against me. I had one hand on each of their backs. Up then down. They were facing each other. Nathaniel had closed his eyes and was almost asleep. The baby girl hadn't opened her eyes yet.

She was beautiful. She looked like me when I was a baby. I had thick black hair at birth and was nearly nine pounds. I even had such round cheeks that my eyes appeared thin. I actually have large round eyes, so I surprised my mother when I opened them for the first time. It's one of the few stories I remember her telling me. She loved her children but didn't know how to care for us. Not like I knew how to care for my children. My grandparents were wonderful parents to my brother and me in her absence.

The little girl startled once in my arms. It made me laugh a little. There was nothing here to startle her, but she jumped anyway. I comforted her by patting her back. She relaxed and drifted away again. I thought about the sun over the trees. What would happen if I didn't get to hold these children while I was awake? How would I give them back to God after spending so much time here with them? I barely knew my daughter, but I loved her. She would be Anastasia Lyn. I pictured a man walking toward us in a white robe. I looked up at the sun. I didn't have to think about that here, not today. Today I was relaxing on the warm beach with two of my children.

I tried to fall asleep with them, but just as I had started to sleep, I heard, Hi Mommy! I looked up. Down the beach across the river were Chloe, Ella and my husband. There was a little fog between us, but I could see Chloe jumping and waving. Ella was looking toward us from Daddy's arms. I waved at Chloe and smiled toward Ryan. I saw him smile. They went back to playing in the sand. They didn't walk down to us in our chair, but I didn't mind. They would probably wake the babies anyway.

~*~

Two

I caught Ella under each arm and picked her up before she ran any further. It's time to get dressed little one. She wrestled with me in her room. I pulled off her pajamas and her soaked diaper. She tucked herself into the corner and pointed down, "butt" she said. She was right, that was a baby butt. I laid her down on her blanket again and tried to get a new diaper on. She was so squirmy! I got the diaper on and she ran off to the living room. I saw Ryan laughing from the dining room table, so I handed him her clothes. "I'll wake up Chloe."

Chloe still looked like a baby in her bed. He arms were always neatly placed under her cheek over her pillow. Her cheeks were still round with baby fat. They had thinned out quite a bit this year, but I could still see it. Her belly stuck out of the bottom of her pajamas. The shirt was crinkled from rolling around all night. I looked at her feet, size 11 in girls'. She was still so little. Her toenails were crooked and filled with grime. The nail polish was flaking off but there were no toe jams. She was diligent about keeping the toe jams from filling the crevices between her toes.

I tickled her back. It's time to wake up Chloe. She wiggled a little but only to shake my hand from her. I rubbed her arm and started to tell her about her day. She had school, then daycare, then home with Mommy. She didn't wake up.

Ella pushed the door open wide and said "Hi, Sissy! Sissy? Sissy!" Chloe rolled over to her and grumbled "Hi, Ella, get out of here." Ella smiled. "Sissy!" Chloe finally sat up and said she was hungry. I pointed her in the direction of the waffles. Before I could catch her Ella army-rolled into Chloe's tent to hide. She was very still but she forgot to pull her foot inside the door. I looked through the window. She was ducking and smiling. Nice try.

I met Ryan at the door of the clinic, and we walked in together. I felt like my belly had grown since the last time I was here. I registered at the desk and snuck into the bathroom. I didn't know if they needed a urine sample, but I didn't think I could wait until I got into the room.

Ryan was reading a popular mechanics magazine when I returned to the lobby to sit by him. I don't think he's interested in mechanics, but it was the only non-female magazine near his chair. I asked him if he was excited. He said he was excited, nervous, and ready. I asked him to pray for me. He said he did. Then he stopped me from looking around to say, whatever happens, this was meant to be. This is what God wants.

I knew that this was meant to happen. I got pregnant while I had an IUD. This was meant to happen. I had confidence when the nurse called my name. We walked together to the scale. I hadn't gained anything since the last time, but it had only been a little over a week. We walked into the ultrasound room where she asked me to get undressed and handed me a paper blanket.

I remembered the ultrasound pictures on the computer a few nights before. How one baby would look and how twins would appear. I remembered the tiny heartbeat and prayed for God to let me see my baby's heart beating.

Ryan looked nervous. He had his hands folded under his chin and was lost in his thoughts. I tried to figure out what he was thinking, but he's hard to read. He looked up and said everything's going to be fine. I knew I was going to be fine, and I knew he would be fine. I was worried about the baby. I knew there was still a chance I had miscarried, but that seemed so long ago already. I still felt pregnant. I took three pregnancy tests since my last visit and they were all still positive. If my HCG levels were going down from 3900, they would have been getting a lighter pink line, not a darker one.

The doctor walked in. He wasn't my regular doctor, but my doctor was not in the office all week. I think they said he was on vacation. This doctor was a little older than mine and instead of family medicine he was certified for obstetrics. I knew he'd do a good job with the ultrasound, but I had one bad experience with him, so I couldn't say I liked him either.

Almost six years earlier I sat in the same room. After he did an ultrasound of Chloe, I told him I was having contractions and they had begun to hurt that morning. He said it was probably gas and that I would be fine. I tried to convince him that I knew the difference, but he didn't believe me. I was 18 and it was my first child. Maybe I didn't know, so I went home.

The pain was getting worse all day, and by 11:30 that night I had to go to the ER. I was sure something was wrong. The same doctor was on call that night, and said I had to take a two-hour ambulance ride to Duluth—the nearest neonatal intensive care unit. I was dilated to three centimeters. I thought he was joking. I even laughed. He didn't. I spent a week in Duluth before I was able to go home. Chloe was almost born at 30 weeks gestation because this doctor told me I was having gas cramps.

I had to trust him. He knew how to do ultrasounds better than anyone else at the clinic. He also seemed to have softened compared to what I remembered. He sat down and told me to lay back. A little cold here. I hated these ultrasounds, but my baby needed me to do this.

The doctor looked around. He studied my uterus and my ovary where almost two weeks ago my doctor pointed out the corpus luteum. He turned the screen so I could see it. He scanned the gestational sac again. Then he measured it for me.

He didn't have to say anything. I could see that it was empty. There was no yolk, or baby. He said the sac was smaller than the last time I had an ultrasound. He said that he was sorry, but that this was a miscarriage. He said he'd give us a minute. I cried. The tears poured from my eyes and my chest felt like something had crushed my ribs. I pushed my face into Ryan's chest. I could hear myself crying and I felt pain with every breath I took in.

~*~

I could hear my weeping in the distance as I stood on the beach looking toward the canopy. They were in there, my babies. I slept with them in my arms on the chair last night. The sun warmed them in my arms. I wasn't crying on the beach. I walked toward the cloth walls stopping short of entering.

~*~

The doctor came back. I was dressed and seated next to Ryan on the bench. He started to explain that what looked like the corpus luteum last time appeared to be a second pregnancy that started within the ovary and grew attached to it.

~*~

I walked into the canopy they were still here. Both children had their eyes open. I picked them up. Nathaniel and Anastasia were both a little heavier today. Maybe they had grown. I fell into the wicker chair and began rocking them. They just looked at each other against my breasts. I should feed them soon.

~*~

The doctor sent Ryan and I over to the hospital to get my HCG levels checked again and made an appointment for later that afternoon. He wanted to go over the results with me in person and what would happen next.

We stepped outside. It was cold, but the sun was out. It felt warm on my neck. We walked along the sidewalk past the flowers in the garden. There were colorful tulips, daffodils, and bushes. Ryan called a colleague to cancel his classes. He held my hand while we walked into the hospital. We had to register there.

Do you want the door closed? Ryan answered for me. I just stared at a message on the wall. Patient rights. I would be provided emergency, stabilizing care even if I could not afford it. Great. She asked me my birthday. It barely squeaked out. I couldn't breathe.

I walked down the hall squeezing Ryan's arm. We sat in the waiting room for the lab. There was a long line of other patients in front of me and they were all staring at me. The woman sitting across from me was a manager at my first job. I was 15. She was sitting with her legs crossed looking at a magazine. She was a nurse now, and through her scrubs I could see her very pregnant belly. She looked at me, but I looked away. I didn't want to say hi. I didn't want to say anything.

Ryan stood up and pulled me out of my chair. He said we were leaving, that I could come back. He knew that sitting there, across from her, was even more depressing than walking out of the doctor's office. I said I had to take the test because I had to come back. Ryan left me in the hallway and walked back to the lab's window. I turned my head into the wall and rested my forehead against it. The wallpaper was awful. The people were still watching me from the crowd around the lab. I didn't want to go back but my baby needed me to.

Ryan came back and said I was next. They lead me to the chair and shut the door. I looked away as she wiped my arm with alcohol and said we'll be out of here in just a second. I squeezed Ryan's hand. "Done."

She asked if I wanted to go out the back door. I said no. Then she addressed Ryan and asked if he wanted to go out the back door. He said yes. We walked past another lab chair and into the radiology office. There you go. The glass doors slid open and we walked out. Ryan gave me a long hug outside under the sun. He walked me to my car. He kissed me then helped me in. The tears wouldn't stop rolling. He walked slowly back to his car where he watched me through the window.

I had to stop the tears before I could drive. Breathe in, breathe out. I wiped the tears from my cheeks. Breathe in breath out. I closed my eyes, turned my head toward the sun, and let the warmth bring me back to the beach.

~*~

We were lying on the quilt in the sand. Ana was on my left and Nathan was on my right. They were both wiggling and studying the beach. Ana was watching the water, then Mommy. Nathan was holding bits of sand in a hand. His eyes were staring right into mine. He was serious. I knew I had to rename them. I never really knew whether they were a boy and a girl. I just felt like they were. I never had to change their diapers either to get a closer look. I didn't need to. Here, it didn't matter.

I opened my eyes to Ryan still watching me from his car. I smiled, waved, started the car and backed out. I should have gone to work like I planned, but instead I met Ryan at a restaurant nearby—Breakwater. I called work to let them know I'd be another half hour. I said I needed to collect myself. It was fine. I'm sure anyone could hear my tears through the phone. I walked into the restaurant as a mother of three.

We sat in the back. The server was very nice to us. I ordered a Diet Pepsi with no ice, and Ryan ordered a coffee. We looked at the menus but decided on sourdough toast. I silently begged him to speak. He could talk about anything, vacation, our house, or our babies. He knew I needed something, so he made a bad joke. At least we have more money for vacation. I laughed. He was still my husband, the man I loved as much as my children.

We should try again. He smiled, we will. We started talking about moving into our new house this summer. Our moving date is July 31st. We talked about where we would put the couch and the rocking chair. Maybe we'd have the two girls in the same room and turn the third bedroom into a playroom. Should we get stools for the backside of the counter? I think they'd fit perfectly.

I stopped at home before returning to work. I needed to put makeup on again and brush my hair. The woman in the mirror was still pregnant. I sat on the couch for a minute. The babies weren't in the sacs we saw on the ultrasound. I thought about the beach.

Ryan, Ella and I piled back into the doctor's office at 3:30. The doctor came in and sat down. He asked if I had any questions. I said no. He began to explain the HCG levels and how they work. He said my test form that morning was over 10,000. I smiled. You mean there is a baby? "No. There is definitely no baby."

He was also sure that the HCG level rising meant that there was another failed pregnancy outside of my uterus, probably in the ovary he'd examined earlier. He needed to do another ultrasound to make sure I wasn't bleeding since that morning. If I was,

I needed surgery right away, if I wasn't, he said it could wait until 6:45 the next morning.

I didn't cry and I didn't drift off to my beach. He asked if I had any questions about the surgery. I did. I asked a lot of questions. After a few minutes of talking I asked if he was sure I'd lost them. He was certain. I agreed to the surgery and took the instruction sheets home.

I didn't cry in the car, and I didn't cry when I got home. I didn't know why I wasn't crying anymore. Maybe I had run out of tears. I was probably in shock. That morning I thought I was going to see a baby's heartbeat but instead I was told I lost two babies and I needed surgery before I started to bleed internally.

I tucked the girls into bed and told Ryan I needed to shower. He said I should wait until morning. I showed him the instructions. They clearly stated to take a shower the night before surgery. I let the water warm up while I stared into the mirror. I was still pregnant. I let my hair down and took my clothes off. I pulled the bobby pins out, and carefully removed my wedding rings, my necklace, my earrings, and my bracelet—all gifts from Ryan.

I removed my garnet ring. My mom had given me that ring when I turned 13. She had her birthstone removed from it and put mine there instead. She received that ring from her dad nearly forty years earlier when she had turned 13. I loved it, and I loved that she had given it to me. I neatly lined everything up on the shelf of the bathroom.

My stomach still didn't hurt. How did I lose my babies without ever feeling any pain? How did I have a pregnancy in my ovary without every feeling it? I thought about the ultrasound. Both gestational sacs were empty. That was comforting. The babies were already gone, so when the doctor removed what was left, they would be spared. They were safe.

I let a few tears fall before I stepped into the water. I let it run until it was very hot. Then I turned it up again. It hurt to put the top of my head under the shower head. I soaked my hair and began rubbing my shampoo into my scalp. I thought about the babies sleeping in their cribs. It was getting dark there. I wanted to be with them, but I had to finish my shower first.

The suds ran down my legs and into the drain. I watched them until they were gone. I took out my razor and began to shave. I didn't feel it against my skin. I wanted to feel it, but I couldn't. I put more soap on after I shaved hoping to feel something, even if it stung. But it didn't.

I used my exfoliating scrub to wash away the salt from the day. Finally, I felt something. It burned. I must have rubbed my face so much with tissue and my rough hands that I had started to pull layers from the surface off. I scrubbed hard to make sure all the oil was removed with my makeup. I would usually wipe all the soap off first and then use a cloth to rinse my face. That time, I plunged my entire face into the running water. The soap ran into my eyes, over my lips and down my neck. My eyes stung with the water touched them; they were already raw from crying. I let the water run across my face for a couple of minutes. I could barely breathe under the water, but I felt that way all day.

I turned the water off and stepped onto the plush rug. I tied my towel around me, and I stood in front of the mirror again. I wanted to be pregnant, but I wasn't anymore. I dried off, put my pajamas on, and crawled into bed. Ryan swung his arm around me and scooted closer. His arm was heavy, but I was comfortable. I could hear the water again.

~*~

Hello there. I smiled and scooped each child into my arms. You two must be hungry. I sat cross legged on the wicker couch and tucked a pillow under each elbow. I turned each wide-eyed child so that their feet were behind me and their noses were positioned just under each of my breasts. There.

They stared at me for a moment, waiting for me to speak. I love you. I sang to them. I didn't know what baby song to sing them, they were perfect. I didn't want them to experience the world that I came from. I sang amazing grace. They listened before my baby girl latched and began to drink. My baby boy followed suit. They were still staring up at me listening. I sang until both of their eyes were closed. I pulled each of their lips, so they'd release me and covered myself. I repositioned each of them so that I had their heads resting on my elbow and their toes touched in my lap.

Goodnight. It was dark on the beach. I could see the moon and stars through the waving cloth walls. The dust was spinning outside, but not much came in where we were sitting. I listened to the water. It seemed to get louder at night without the birds singing. I didn't want to fall asleep. I wanted to soak in every second I had with my babies. I thought about when I'd have to hand them to the man in the white robe. I would when I had to, but I wasn't ready yet. I was still caring for them, and we were doing well.

~*~

Morning finally crept in through the curtains. I walked to the window to look out. Frost. I put on my best sweatpants, Ryan's sweatshirt, and I brushed my hair. I walked to the bathroom to brush my teeth. I sat to use the toilet and looked down. I was bleeding. The doctor was right, my babies were gone. I couldn't flush. I walked away before I realized Chloe might see. I went back to flush and watched the blood swirl before it disappeared.

Three

The parking lot only had two other cars in it. The employees must park in the back. I took a deep breath in. I had to let the doctor remove what was left of my pregnancies. I walked in to register. My surgery appointment wasn't even in the computer yet. I didn't have a chart, or an assigned bed. The nurse explained that I was an add-on for first of the day.

I waited for Ryan. They asked me to take off my clothes; everything but my socks. I had a purple gown that covered everything when it was tied—the ends overlapped. There were paw prints on the front of it. It looked silly with my black socks.

The nurse asked me the required questions. Why are you here today? I had a heterotopic pregnancy, I lost both, and I have to have the ectopic pregnancy removed. The doctor said he may have to remove part of my ovary. She looked sad but didn't say anything. I told her I had two other daughters. She told me the doctor and the anesthesia nurse would be in to see me before they took me into to operating room.

My doctor came first. He went over all of the parts of the procedure again and explained why he had to do it. I asked one more time if he was sure that the babies were already gone. He was sure.

The anesthesiologist came next and explained how I would first be given something in my IV to relax, and then they would put the breathing mask over my mouth to finish putting me to sleep. I didn't like it. I asked how long it would take to wake up. He laughed and said I would wake up within 5 minutes of completing the surgery, but probably wouldn't remember anything for another 20 minutes. The nurse said that some patients were combative during the first 20 minutes when they weren't fully aware of their surroundings.

Just as the surgical nurse came over to introduce herself to me, I heard Ryan's voice. He walked in and hugged me. He said that my gown looks like the ones from his veterinarian's office. The nurse explained that in just a minute they'd start my IV then take me into the operating room. I cringed when she said IV. She said they'd numb my arm first.

I watched the nurse organizing the tray until I realized she'd picked up a needle. I turned away and covered my eyes. Ryan came over to rub my leg. Just a pinch and a little burn. I should not be so afraid of needles, but I can't help it. It's worse if I try to watch. I only felt the IV going in a little, barely enough to cringe but I did that anyway.

Ok we're all set. Ryan came over to give me a warm hug and kissed me. I hugged him one more time and kissed his neck. I love you.

The room was tile from the floor to the ceiling. Directly over my bed the ceiling was made of metal ceiling tile. There was a large hanging light over me they turned on. It reminded me of the dentist's office. Ok, we're going to give you something to relax. I was dizzy right away and started to laugh.

That was it. I don't remember anything until the recovery room. I don't remember the mask, or the doctors. I know what they did, but I don't remember any of it. I felt warm and cozy when I woke up. I asked the nurse how things went. She said they went well. I fell back to sleep. I think I was in a different room than before. But when I opened my eyes again, I was in my room with Ryan.

How did it go? Ryan said everything went well and that they removed my right ovary. Will the other one still work? The nurse smiled and said yes. I didn't see the doctor again that day. They said I'd see him on Thursday, 6 days later. I wanted to know if he was right, if it was a second pregnancy. I needed to ask him if I could still have children. I wanted to know if I bled, or if everything went smoothly. The nurse said I could talk to him on Thursday.

She pulled me up to sitting. I had to walk around a little before I could go home. I took a second to steady my head before I stood up on the floor. Blood rushed down my legs and onto the tile floor. I'm so sorry. I started crying. I'm so sorry. The nurse tried to calm me telling me that it was OK. I asked to sit back down. She handed me a towel to wipe my legs off. Another nurse came with a warm washcloth to help. It hurt to lean forward.

I need my clothing bag. It has my underwear and my pads in it. She offered the hospital net underwear for me, but I told her mine would be fine. She came back with it and I carefully attached the thick pad and slid them on. More blood made it down my leg. I grabbed the warm cloth and cleaned it off again fighting the tears.

I tried to wipe the floor up, but the nurse pulled me back up telling me I couldn't bend over that way for a while. She and Ryan helped me walk to the bathroom. She said I should try to go. I sat down and waited. It took a while before I was able to pee. When the stream ended, I could still hear dripping. I looked down and there was more blood. I was still bleeding. I stood, cleaned myself up with a towel, and pulled the string on the wall. The nurse came back and helped me back to the bed. Before I sat down, I saw the large blood stain I had made. I'm so sorry.

When it was time to leave, I sat up again. I had a hard time breathing this time. I told the nurse that I thought I was panicking. She said it was the air leftover form the laparoscopy migrating to my shoulders. That it was completely normal to have my breath taken away for a couple of hours after surgery. She was right, my shoulders, neck, and stomach really hurt. She said the doctor had left a prescription for oxycodone.

Ryan drove me home and I laid on the couch right away. I didn't know if my beach would still be there, or if it would still be dark. I imagined my piano dancing over the canopy for my babies. I thought about what I would name them now that I didn't know whether they were boys or girls. As I drifted off, I decided I would find unisex names, so it wouldn't matter when I wrote it down; just like it didn't matter at the beach.

~*~

The sun was warm again on my back. I walked toward the canopy. There they were awake, waiting for Mommy. I stepped out for a second to pull the blanket into the shade behind the canopy. I picked them up and set them onto the blanket next to each other. They were watching me. I began to sing about them. I sang about their toes, their fingers, their bellies. I held their hands and kissed their heads. I even brushed their hair from their foreheads for them. They were so beautiful.

~*~

Ella was climbing onto the couch when I opened my eyes. Hi, Mommy! Hi, Pumpkin. Chloe was busy playing in her room. I asked Ryan to take Ella so she wouldn't hurt me. It was almost dinner time; I had slept all day. I carefully stood and walked to the bathroom.

I pulled my shirt up. My stomach was orange with iodine. I had two small bandages with dried blood visible from each side and one large bandage across my belly button. The large bandage had blood soaked through it. There were definitely no babies in my belly now. I tried not to cry, but I'm not sure I could have even if I tried.

Ryan asked how I slept. Fine. I didn't know what to say. I asked him how he was. Fine. I wasn't sure if losing the babies even bothered him. It must have. He was probably just trying to be strong for me. At least it made me feel better to believe that.

Dinner was uncomfortable. Ryan did his best to make me happy. He chose foods I loved—fried chicken, macaroni and cheese, mashed potatoes (for him), and peas. I wasn't hungry. Chloe asked how my day was. It was long. Why was it long? Because mommy had to go to the doctor's today. Why? Because I needed to have surgery. Why? Just because. I couldn't break her heart. I didn't even want mine to break this way.

Ryan tried to have fun with the girls. He made faces at Ella and asked for details about Chloe's day. Chloe didn't usually like to share the details of her day. But she could see something was wrong with Mommy, so she went into her story. She'd been dropped off by grandma, she wasn't late, and she played outside with her friends. One of them isn't her friend anymore because she was being mean. She also had music class and would like to sing her new song to us. What's the rule, Chloe? No singing at the dinner table. Her eyes rolled up when she said it. I promised I'd listen after dinner.

Ryan tried to play a movie for everyone after dinner. I excused myself to go to bed. He watched me walk until I disappeared down the hallway. How could I watch a movie after this?

My bed was still messy from the morning. I pulled the comforter off and tidied the sheet. The comforter was heavier today. I swung my arms up to spread it across the sheet, and then tightened the wrinkles out of the surface. I folded the blankets back and crawled in. They were cold. I turned my iPod on to my relaxing music. I was so tired, but I just needed a minute with them.

~*~

The sky was brighter today, and the air was a bit cooler than I remembered. There were purple glowing clouds over the water. The lake was dull. There weren't many waves but the ones that rolled in barely wet the rocks they touched. The sun was just under the rolling hills to the East. Maybe the water would gleam again when the sun peered over the hill.

The canopy walls waved in the wind. I could still see the cribs and the wicker furniture when they flapped back. I was afraid to go in. My chair still sat along the edge of the sand, and the blanket was still lying behind the canopy with wrinkles from our bodies resting on it.

I didn't know if I could go in. I prayed that they'd still be there. I didn't want them to be cold. Did they have blankets? I walked slowly to the opening letting my feet drag through the sand. They were sleeping. They each had their blanket wrapped around them snugly. I looked down to my baby with light hair. I kneeled next to his crib and looked through the wooden bars. His breath was so soft. His chest rose up and down. I walked over to the second crib. There was my baby. Her face was angled toward me slightly. She looked so tired. I didn't think I could wake them up; they were sleeping so sound. I lay near them on the wicker couch. I folded the pillow to make it a little higher and pulled the knitted blanket over my shoulders. I pulled my toes up under the blanket and trapped it under my feet. My eyes checked the babies one more time before they closed. The water seemed so far away from inside.

~*~

Sunday morning, we packed the girls up in the car and took them to the park. They loved the park. Ella was not afraid of the tall slides. Sometimes we'd have to jump to catch her before she went down without her feet first.

We didn't catch her once. Ryan was almost at the top of the platform. One of her feet was stuck under her little diaper butt when she started to slide down. She twisted and looked to Mommy to help. I couldn't reach her yet. At the halfway point she tried to pull her leg out and fell back hitting her head against the hard-blue plastic. I caught her at the bottom. She was already screaming. It happened so fast, but I remember every detail. She clung to me so tightly while she cried. I just hugged her, bounced, and turned in circles. Just like when she was a baby.

We are always told not to react when a child gets hurt. But I couldn't help but hold her while she cried. She only cried for a few minutes. Then she heard Chloe yell for us to watch her. She looked up at Sissy and from behind her tears still trapped on her lid, she smiled. Her wet, dirty face was precious. She started to wriggle to get down. I gave her one more kiss and set her on the wood chips. She ran away.

Today was different. She was a little bigger now and nearly immune to head bumps and falls. Running to the big jungle gym she tripped over her feet and went face first into the wood chips and dirt. She stood up, spit out the dirt, and wiped her hands on her Daddy as he tried to pick her up. She ran toward the stairs instead.

Chloe only liked to play on the pieces that we were not playing on. When we pack the girls up in the car for a trip to the park, we imagine a fun, exciting time with the four of us playing together, swinging together, and having our snack together. Our ideas are always shattered as Chloe runs one way and Ella goes another. Ryan and I just waved from the opposite sides of the city block sized park.

After the park we relaxed at home with a snack. The girls love the tiny cheese flavored cracker in the shapes of bunnies and fish. They didn't talk much during snack, they were so tired. Chloe said she was going to watch television in our room. We knew she'd fall asleep, so we said yes. Ella cried to get down after a couple of bites, so I held her in my arms like a newborn baby, handed her the bottle, and walked her into her dark bedroom.

She smiled up at me and put her finger to my nose. I put mine to hers. Sleep well, tiny girl. I love you. I set her gently onto her mattress while she stared up at me from behind her bottle. Her little fingers were sticky with dirt in the creases. She is perfect. I leaned over the railing one more time to fix her blanket for her. A twinge crept up my spine starting at my belly button. I jumped a little. I blew a kiss to Ella as I slowly shut the door.

I walked down the hall to check on Chloe. The floor was covered in play dishes, Little People, and dress up clothes. I peeked through the crack into our bedroom. Chloe was already asleep. Her little back was arched with her belly button sticking out of her shirt. She had her hands folded under her cheek and dirt lines across her face. I smiled. *Dirt just means she had a good time at the park.*

Monday, I stayed home from work. I smiled while I got the girls ready for school and day care. I kissed Ryan goodbye and locked the door behind them. I stood in the empty house. I thought about the girls I loved, my sweet husband, and my babies on the beach. The tears fell, hard. This time, I let them fall. I didn't lie in my bed and wait for the sun or smile because my girls were watching. I let myself cry.

I wandered through the house looking at the mess of toys and school papers. I thought about how my two babies wouldn't get to go to school or know how much I loved them. I worried that the girls should know, so they could love them too, but that I couldn't tell them until they were older. I thought about the attic at the new house, and how we could take our time to finish it into a bedroom. Maybe we could just make it a playroom, or leave it as an attic. I sat in the rocking chair and stared at the overgrown grass and the apple blossoms. I just needed to cry.

Lunch came around and I searched the cabinets in the kitchen. I had packets of rice, cookies, frozen vegetables, and leftovers. I thought about eating something, but I couldn't. I poured myself a diet Pepsi. I decided it was time to take a nap. I took off my clothes, tied my hair back, and fell into bed. The tears came again when I stared from my room to the hallway. I should clean that up. But instead, my eyelids grew heavier.

~*~

The sun was warm on my face. My cheeks were still wet from my bed, but the sun began to dry them. The babies were sleeping in their beds. I picked them up and carried them to our chair. Each child slept on my shoulders. I could feel their moist breath on my skin. I stared off into the waves where the sun was weaving through the edge of every crest. The blanket lay gently over the children's backs, protecting them from the sun, and I pulled my hat down a little further to shield my eyes. I let them sleep and let my eyes close under the sun.

That night went well. I greeted my family at the door and made dinner with Ryan. We talked about each other's days and had ice cream together. I tucked the girls in and watched TV with my husband. I felt sad, but happy at the same time. I decided I'd try to go to work the next day.

~*~

The shower was hot when I got in the next morning. It

burned a little, so I turned the heat down. Ella followed me as her daddy tried to peel her pajamas off before she soaked them. Butt! She knew all her body parts and showed them off when she was bare. Button! He looked so tiny in our shower, but she played like we were in our swimsuits at the beach. She grabbed the old washcloths that were collecting in the corner, and rubbed sop onto her belly and arms. Toes! I let her wash my toes in the water. She wanted to help.

I called for Ryan to grab her towel before I turned the water off; I didn't want her to get cold. He pulled the towel out and wrapped her up in it. She shivered while she cried to rejoin me. I turned the water off, wiped my face, and stepped onto the carpet. I can do this.

Chloe and Ryan ran out the door just in time for the bus driver to see them and stop. She laughed as they crossed the street; she loved the excitement of the last minute. Ryan waved to the driver and the bus was off again. Ella was watching cartoons in the rocking chair. Ryan and I finished getting ready and packed up the bags. Ella was going to ride with me to day care.

When we arrived, I pulled her out of the car and swung her bags around my shoulder. She held my hand as we walked together to the door. The other kids were hopping out of their cars with their parents, too. I watched to make sure Ella was out of the way as the door closed behind her. She knew which room was hers, the toddler room. I lifted her over the gate, and she waited for me to come in. She held onto my leg as I walked to her hook. I knelt beside her and asked if she wanted to play. She nodded a very clear yes. I hugged her and she walked to her friends. I took one more look before I waved and left. She didn't see me.

As I drove to work, I started to cry. I'd never drop my babies off at daycare or kiss them goodbye. I would never get to tuck them in at night or play on the floor. I could barely see as I drove. I walked in to thank one of our corporate employees for coming to cover me while I was out. She hugged me and said they were in heaven now. I pictured them on our beach. I thanked my boss for his help and taking care of everything so I could be out for a few days. I was wearing business clothing but explained that I couldn't stay. I wanted to try but I couldn't. I told them I'd try again tomorrow.

Waves of sadness rolled over me as I drove down the street toward my house. I waited at the stop sign for a second to wipe the tears away. I could see our mailbox from that corner. The driveway was empty, and the dandelions had taken over the yard. I stopped at the next stop sign. A car or two passed and I rolled onto my block. I drove slowly. I didn't know if I should keep driving or stop. I stopped; I couldn't see where I was going anyway.

~*~

I had my appointment the next morning with the doctor. I had so many questions for him. As I crawled into bed, I knew I needed to spend the night on the beach with my babies. I let the sun beat on my back while I walked to the canopy. I picked them up as I had so many times before and walked out to our chair. I laid back and let them sleep on my chest. I didn't cover them this time. They needed a little sun. There were dark curls on my left, and light straight strands of hair tickling my neck on my right.

I wanted to paint this moment. I wanted the painting to show me looking down at the children's hands lying perfectly over the center of my chest, their fingers touching. I wanted my hat to shield my eyes, and each child to look so alive that the viewer could see their breathing through the paint. I pictured the air a little foggy, and the sand to look cool enough to lie on without the blanket. I wanted the waves to be near the shore but the sparkling rocks to be visible through the fog as their eyes follow the shoreline. There would be the river between us and the silhouettes of Ryan and our two little girls in the distance.

The trees behind us would be brilliant green and turn grey as they faded into the cloud. There would be a piercing sun and visible rays touching us all slightly different shades of color. The white blanket would be pure white. And beneath the edge there would be baby toes resting comfortably against my skin. I'd have a hand over each of their backs. The painting would be perfect in the center of our living room.

~*~

I rolled out of bed while it was still quiet. Ryan had already run. He said it was cold out. I was quiet. I wandered through the house waiting for the right time to wake the girls. I showered, dressed, and sat on the edge of Chloe's bed. I did the "tickle walk" on her back. My two fingers would walk up her back—she said that it tickled but she loved it. She groaned and turned; she pulled her blanket up to her head and tried to kick me. I told her she had to go to school. She wouldn't get up.

Ryan must have let Ella out of her bed because she charged into the room. Hi, Sissy! Chloe smiled and opened her eyes. Hi, Ella. She sat up and tickled Ella. I asked if they were hungry and they screamed yes. Choc-at! Choc-at! Ella wasn't going to get chocolate for breakfast, but I waited to tell her until after I had her buckled into her chair. Cute little girls.

The clinic seemed empty. It was 11:15 when I walked in, but it seemed dead. There was only one other person in the waiting room. I checked-in with the registration desk. The man sitting there remembered my name and that I had recently been in. He said I was all set before I even sat down. I thanked him and waited for someone to say my name.

Next to me there was a woman slightly older than me with a tiny newborn. He slept wrapped in his animal blanket. His mom rocked him with her toe while she filled out check to pay her bills. A nurse appeared around the corner and said her name. She laughed when she saw the checkbook. Multi-tasking? They smiled as they walked through the doors to the next room.

I tried to think of anything else, but my questions played over and over in my head. Were there really two? Did the IUD leave damage? When can I get pregnant again? I couldn't relax. I heard my name and it startled me. I tried to smile at the nurse. She remembered me too. She smiled but I knew she felt bad for me. I tried to make a joke about my two naughty girls at home. But her expression remained the same.

I let her check my oxygen, blood pressure, and heart rate. The doctor will be right in. She silently escaped through the door. I sat in the office looking at the walls. On the back of the door there was an ad for a different type of IUD. It was a permanent form of birth control. Irreversible. The calendar featured photographs of grassy fields with wildflowers. The magazine rack was filled with parenting magazines, a Reader's Digest, and WebMD's magazine.

Behind me was a poster showing every month of pregnancy. I stood to look at it. At one month it was still a dot floating around. At two there was a sack, a baby, and a yolk visible. I had never seen my babies or the yolk. Only the sac. I flopped back onto the plastic covered bench. There were drawers next to me filled with coloring books and crayons—Ella would love them.

The doctor came in and asked if I had questions. I let them all pour out of me. He should have been confused or he should have lost some as they tumbled. But he was composed, and calm. He began by explaining that the surgery went well. He said that my levels should start coming down again, and that we'd check them that day. He said that the pregnancy within my uterus has already begun to deteriorate based on the lab report.

I asked about the second pregnancy. It wasn't a pregnancy at all. It was some type of benign adenoma 6 centimeters wide. It had its own fluid, and blood supply, but it was not cancerous. It's why he removed my ovary. He explained that I was at a slightly higher risk to develop more of these tumors than other women. I thought about losing my other ovary. Can I run again, and have sex? "Yep, you can have as much fun and exercise as you'd like."

What are you going to do about birth control? I said we were going to try again right away. I really didn't know if we were, but I wasn't going to have another IUD put in. He thought for a second and said. "You could right away, but it's not about your physical self. It's when you're ready up here and here." He pointed to his head, and his heart. I nodded. He was right. I had no idea what I'd do about more children. Thank you. I shook his hand and he was gone.

I walked to my car and sat for a minute staring through the windshield. The bluffs were visible in the distance. I could see the cars driving past me through my rear-view mirror, and the people walking in and out of the clinic. There was only one baby, I'd only lost one. I wondered who the other baby was on the beach. Was that baby coming next? Did that baby already come and go; I lost it without knowing? I decided that my children were Gabriel Lyn List, and Shiloh Silas List. Maybe the babies were just in my imagination. My way of understanding what happened, and how I felt most comfortable loving something I'd never seen or planned. I didn't know what to think. I started my car and drove back to work.

My iPod played a workout mix. All the songs were fast and full of energy and rhythm. I felt my heart pumping fast, my arms and legs moving rhythmically, and my feet pounding into the blacktop. The hill was long. The road came to a T and I turned right. I always did the entire hill—Mount Zion.

I didn't run up the hill because it was a great workout, or because there was anything at the top waiting for me. It wasn't a shortcut either. I ran up the hill because the light was magnificent.

The bottom of the hill was partially shaded by the trees now that the leaves were fully grown. There was a deep ditch with water at the bottom. The water that was left would dry out soon leaving soft mud. Halfway up the hill I passed an abandoned brick building. It still stood heavily on the side of the bluff, clean, and intact. It was just empty.

As I approached the last part of the hill the trees enclosed over me and the road became dark. The blacktop was old and beginning to crumble at its edges. There was broken glass sparkling in the specks of light that trickled through the leaves.

The peak wasn't any lighter. It was still shaded. I felt a rush of relief as I began running down the hill. The leaves thinned as I ran. I felt the sun growing warmer on my face eventually spilling over the treetops and all over my skin.

I looked up at the sun running alongside of me. I remembered this sun at my beach, my wedding, and on the sidewalk at the hospital. I thought of the park and the girls running away from us to the jungle gym and swings. I thought of Ryan waiting for me at home. I smiled as I ran. I felt the sweat dripping down skin, my hair swinging, and my feet pushing off the road. I ran six miles that day, but I was almost home.